The Gift
of Receiving

Release the Shame and Guilt that
Hold You Back from a Rich
and Delicious Life

Moira Lethbridge, M.Ed.

ISBN 978-1-936961-49-8

Cover and sketches by Madison Hubbard

Art by Marylou Falstreau

Published by LINX
LINX, Corp.
Box 613
Great Falls, VA 22066
www.linxcorp.com

Printed in the United States of America

Dedication

*To my Angel Tribe—Gail and Tammy—who guide me
on this amazing journey and encourage me
to let my light shine.*

Acknowledgements

I would like to thank Cate Pearce for her help in telling this story, who has been my assistant and friend for almost two years. I respect her talents and am grateful to receive her gift of bringing my innermost thoughts to life.

Table of Contents

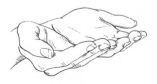

CHAPTER 1
Crashing Expectations

"Did you hit the button on the coffee machine yet?" she mumbled. Her kids were screaming, "It's Christmas! Get up, get up!" One eye opened to see the time: 5:23 a.m.

Coffee mug in one hand and camera in the other, Eileen settled into her chair. Controlled chaos. A blur of wrapping paper, squeals, and crashing expectations. Cinnamon rolls and chocolate. Caffeine and gratitude warmed her body and soul.

Gifts she had bought for the boys covered the floor, everything that they had asked for on their Christmas lists that she could afford.

"Mom, what about your Christmas presents? Where did Santa hide them?" Tony asked, his attention occupied by the toy truck in his hands.

1

"Santa gave all of Mommy's gifts to you guys this year." Eileen smiled, more than happy to have sacrificed any money for the boys rather than get herself things she didn't need (and probably didn't deserve). She had already spent enough money getting her car fixed after she accidentally backed into a fence on a stressful morning commute to work.

Tony shrugged and all three boys returned to their Christmas reverie, their gifts sure to keep them occupied until they went to their dad's house later.

***

"You can only bring one toy to Dad's house. That's the rule."

Eileen scampered from room to room, packed overnight bags, favorite pillows and blankets, and put the dog in the crate. The kids slept on the drive to her former husband's house, and she only stayed for enough time to get the kids settled before she started the drive home, wanting to avoid spending any more time than necessary with her ex. She changed the radio station from the music the boys liked to a random self-help podcast, one that promised to "restore the light in women's eyes." The lesson fell on deaf ears, but it stopped the tears dropping from Eileen's eyes and filled up the silence that the boys' absence created.

CHAPTER 1

Eileen returned home and sank to her knees, no strength left to stand. Desolate sobs. Being alone and away from her children left her feeling intense anguish. Her body drained, she climbed into bed and slept, resigned to spending her Christmas alone and miserable. She didn't deserve anything more.

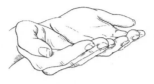

CHAPTER 2
Separation Anxiety

Eileen gulped her smoothie as she scanned the highway for cops. The voice in her head droned on, *You're late again. You're always late. You're not doing it right.* Her chest and head pounded. *I can make it on time.* She pulled into a parking spot with two minutes to spare. Eileen brushed her hair with her hand, pasted on a smile, and greeted Lizzy.

"I can't believe it. You made it on time!" Lizzy's eyes sparkled, her arms open and expecting a hug from her longtime friend. Eileen fell into it, feeling the love and gentleness that always shone from Lizzy.

"It's so nice to see you, Eileen," Noella said, standing behind Lizzy and hugging Eileen as well. Noella had been traveling, and this was the first time the three friends had been together in the same place for a long time. Eileen couldn't help but feel jealous of Noella's wanderings, as she wished she could live that kind of life.

"This restaurant looks great!" Lizzy said. "Thanks for finding it, Eileen."

"Oh, I didn't do anything more than Google 'nice Greek food.' A monkey could've done it," Eileen responded as the three women walked into the front lobby and were seated.

"I don't know if I'm going to be able to go to Portugal with you, Noella," Eileen muttered demurely, already feeling the pushback her friends were about to give her.

"What do you mean? I thought we already had it figured out," Noella softly asked, her brown eyes crinkling in worry, or maybe disappointment, in Eileen.

"Well, I can't just leave the boys for weeks to fend for themselves. And the dog has been going through a lot of separation anxiety lately, not to mention I have to keep up with my business and figure out how to get more clients. In fact, this would be the worst possible time to go galivanting around the world."

Lizzy sighed and slumped farther in her chair.

"Are you listening to me?" Eileen barked.

CHAPTER 2

"Of course I am. It's just that you've told me a million reasons why you can't say yes to this opportunity, and it's wearing me down."

Eileen's face went ashen. She sighed as her eyes stung with tears. "I want to go, but I miss my husband. My world was turned upside down when he left me. I want my old life back."

"I know you're grieving. But it's been a year, and you're still saying the same exact things you did the day after the breakup. You'd rather blame your ex-husband than admit you're afraid to try something new."

Noella rolled her fork between her fingers, having decided what to say. "Eileen, we travel really well together. I want you to go with me to Portugal for a month as my guest. Please say yes."

Eileen rubbed her forehead to make the pain behind it go away. "I can't."

"Why not?" Lizzy snapped.

"It's not practical. I need to be available for my sons. Who will take care of my dog? What if something bad happens?"

"Your ex-husband has already said yes to taking the boys and the dog. He knows how to dial 911. And of course you feel guilty for going away," said Lizzy. "You've never allowed yourself to catch a break, let alone go after something you really want."

"I can't just leave my business to go off and play."

"You're not going off and 'playing.' You are going after what you want. You already meet with most of your customers online."

"It's just not realistic, Lizzy."

Lizzy rolled her eyes and sat back in her chair. "You really love to punish yourself, Eileen. You believe that it's all up to you, that you have to make it happen, that you are completely independent and strong and have to prove it to everyone. Your compulsion to do everything yourself is killing you."

"It's not a compulsion!" Eileen argued.

Tears stung Eileen's eyes as she fumbled for a crumpled Kleenex in her purse. An intense pressure covered her chest.

Eileen whispered, "I don't know how to stop doing what I've always done. I've never strayed from the path, from the expectation that I support my family at all costs. How can I support my family if I'm not with them? What will people say about me when I tell them I'm leaving my kids to live in a small European town for a month? And my clients might not stay with me if they learn that I'd rather take a vacation than help them. What if it all comes crashing down . . . "

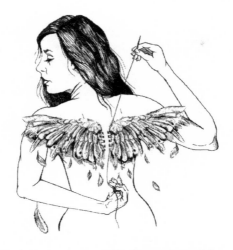

"You don't have to carry all the responsibility yourself. You have options," Noella said after Eileen's words hung in the air for a couple moments.

Eileen grumbled.

Noella continued, "What if you gave yourself permission to do this? What would you do? How would it look? How would you feel?"

"I would go and enjoy every second of it."

"Terrific! See—you can do this. Write down the pros and cons of saying yes to this gift and see which list is longer."

Eileen slumped in her chair. *This is too much.*

"Ugh," she groaned. "My mind doesn't work that way. I draw pictures to make sense of things." *Why bother,* she thought. *It won't make any difference. Noella doesn't understand.*

"Then draw away and see what happens," suggested Noella.

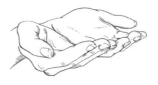

CHAPTER 3
Memories of Crayons

Eileen sat down at the desk in her office. *How long has it been since I doodled*, she wondered. Years certainly. Memories started flashing through her mind, of hours spent with crayons and colored pencils, creating images from her mind's eye. She remembered TIG, an imaginary friend who had been in Eileen's life since she was a child. They'd had lots of fun drawing and talking together. TIG helped her through her crazy childhood. Eileen eventually lost touch with TIG because of her belief that drawing and being creative weren't productive.

Where is that sketchbook? The closet or attic? Eileen rummaged through the guest room closet. It was stuffed with winter coats, sports equipment, and storage boxes. There it was—"MOM'S JUNK" scribbled on the outside of a tattered banker box.

Eileen pulled out her childhood sketchbook. She was transported back in time as she looked at her old drawings. Her heart twinged. Her body buzzed. She started to draw.

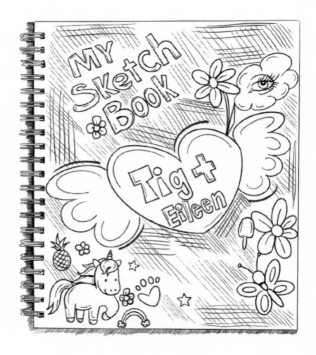

Eileen sketched out her thoughts and beliefs.

"This castle is my home. It's where I live with my dog, my sons, and where I work. If I go to Portugal for a month and leave my castle, will I be OK?"

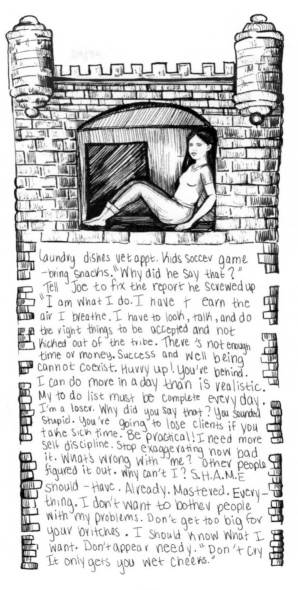

Laundry dishes vet appt. Kids soccer game — bring snacks. "Why did he say that?" Tell Joe to fix the report he screwed up. "I am what I do. I have t earn the air I breathe. I have to look, talk, and do the right things to be accepted and not kicked out of the tribe. There's not enough time or money. Success and well being cannot coexist. Hurry up! You're behind. I can do more in a day than is realistic. My to do list must be complete every day. I'm a loser. Why did you say that? You sounded stupid. You're going to lose clients if you take sick time. Be practical! I need more self discipline. Stop exaggerating how bad it. What's wrong with me? Other people figured it out. Why can't I? S.H.A.M.E should - have. Already. Mastered. Every- thing. I don't want to bother people with my problems. Don't get too big for your britches. I should know what I want. Don't appear needy." Don't cry It only gets you wet cheeks."

13

As her pen worked around the page, the ink following her movement, Eileen started to remember more details about TIG: her pink hair and bewildering mix of a punk rocker and rag doll. Eileen increasingly felt TIG reemerge from the depths of her long-term memory, until it seemed almost as if TIG was sitting right next to her.

"It's been a long time, Leenie," TIG said. Eileen jumped, frightened at the sudden presence of her childhood friend.

"TIG?! How is this possible? I'm too old to have imaginary friends," Eileen cried, wondering if she'd finally crossed the line into insanity.

"I've been here, you just forgot about me for a while," TIG shrugged. "What's making you so upset right now?"

"This Portugal trip . . . the divorce . . . the business . . . everything." The tears poured out of her.

"Well. Let's try to figure this out, one step at a time. What would you do if you won the lottery today?"

"I would sleep—a lot more."

"Great," said TIG. "After you are well rested, tell me all the things you would do in Portugal."

Eileen returned to drawing and froze. Her shoulders caved in on themselves and her head dropped to her desk in a heap, inspiration and drawing abandoned. "There's no way this will work."

"What bad could happen by allowing yourself to be happy?"

"Other people will judge me as irresponsible. They'll think I'm lazy, cheating, doing it wrong, cutting corners. I won't make enough money if I spend time traveling. I'm supposed to be making money. That's what other people are doing. And if I'm successful, that's even worse."

"What happens if you're successful?"

Her pasty face told the truth.

"People will leave me."

"You're afraid to let your light shine," said TIG. "You keep yourself in that castle so nobody can hurt you. Or abandon you. Except that's not what happens; castles can't protect you from life. Go on this trip."

"Why?" asked Eileen.

"Because you have the brightest light, which makes it easier for others to see. Give yourself permission and go. I'm here for you, Eileen. Trust the process. I've got your back."

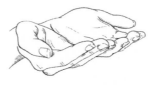

CHAPTER 4

If Nothing Changes,
Nothing Changes

Eileen rushed back into her office, struggling to get the remnants of her nonfat soy latte out of her silk blouse before she had to Zoom with one of her clients.

"Why do these things always have to happen to me?," she muttered, resigned to her fate. She didn't even have enough energy to fuel her busy morning. Tide stick in hand, she sat down at her desk and opened her laptop, noting the time: three minutes until she had to initiate the video call.

In the upper right corner of her computer, she received a notification for one of her daily meditation emails, which she usually disregarded completely. Something about this one made her examine the subject line: *"It's time to stop thinking you should be someone other than who you are, wanting something other than what you really want, and doing something other than what you want to be doing."* Eileen glanced at her old sketchbook, covered in hearts and color.

She needed to go to Portugal.

The stain on her blouse mocked her. "Who do you think you are? You can't even drink without spilling on your nice shirt. You're pathetic."

Eileen clicked on the Zoom icon. The spinning pinwheel mocked her. "Nothing is going to happen until I say it's going to happen."

"God dammit! Now I'm late for my client session."

"Force quit the offending application and start again," TIG whispered.

As she waited for Zoom to restart, she texted her client. "Sorry—technical difficulties. Be there in 5." Eileen hated being late for anything. As a life coach, she knew that shit happened and tried to roll with the punches. But not today.

Eileen's face flushed. Blood pooled in her stomach and a tinny taste flooded her mouth. She glared at the text and picture that just came in from her ex. "Having fun with the boys at Six Flags!"

Her fisted hands pounded her thighs. "Screw it all to hell!"

Eileen texted Noella. "I'm going."

Noella texted back. "Terrific!"

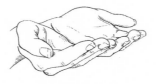

CHAPTER 5
The Thing

"The boys are going to stay with their father, and the dog too," Eileen answered.

"OK, what about the house?" Lizzy asked while she checked a box on the "How To Get To Portugal" to-do list in front of her.

"One of my clients has a daughter who's home from college. I can see if she would be willing to house-sit?" Eileen posited, walking over to Lizzy at the kitchen table with two mugs of tea.

"Perfect!" Lizzy exclaimed, marking another box off.

"What if that's too much, though? Asking her to live in my house for a month? I don't even know what I would have to pay her. What if she has friends over for a party?"

Eileen fussed with her napkin.

"If you know the daughter and the mother, why would you need to worry? It doesn't hurt to ask, and I'm sure the girl would be happy to get any extra cash," Lizzy explained.

Eileen exhaled sharply; the idea of asking a client for help hurt her brain. She was the one who helped other people.

"You're right." Eileen relented. "It's OK to ask people for help. I'll text my client today and see what she says," The admission immediately set her at ease, the growing pains of opening up to the world again reminded her that she was evolving.

Lizzy left after a little bit and Eileen, alone in her house again, went into her office and sat at her desk. She reached for her sketchbook, took out her favorite pen and started to doodle on a blank page. Trying to channel her feelings from earlier, the growing pains and the heartache of trying to get to Portugal, a figure starts to emerge on the canvas. Reminiscent of The Blob from the movie of the same name, Eileen's pen created a Thing, messy and dark and twisted, while her heart started to beat faster and faster and her hands started to shake and sweat. Her body went into defense mode, an evolutionary response to bears and tigers in the woods, which in modern days was described as a panic attack.

ICK.

All of Eileen's negative thoughts and beliefs, self-doubt, guilt, and shame manifested in one being. ICK's voice kept pounding in her head: "Time is money. Don't waste time. You're behind. What you want doesn't matter. Being creative is stupid. You're only good for meeting other people's needs. Stop being so selfish. Keep your priorities straight. You're going to regret this decision."

Eileen slumped in her chair. She whispered, "I'm sorry" to nobody.

"You're so unreasonable. If Noella finds out the truth about you, she'll send you packing," ICK shouted.

Eileen gasped for air, dropping her pen as she tried to calm down. All of her fears and worries personified into a Thing.

She took a minute to consider her drawing, feeling her heartbeat slowing down. "Well, now at least I know what I have to deal with to get better."

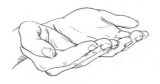

CHAPTER 6
Donning Armor

Her alarm clock blaring, Eileen got out of bed and finished the last of her packing. Again, the nerves started to rise up in her. As excited as she was to be in Portugal the next day, she still felt the doubt; she felt so selfish.

But something within her arose: *It's OK. Everything's going to be OK.*

Eileen grabbed the handle of her suitcase, knowing that her taxi to the airport was outside, and locked the front door of her house.

"What the heck is that?" asked TIG.

Eileen's armor sparkled in the daylight.

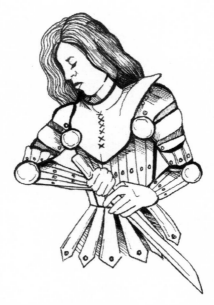

"It's my portable castle. It will keep me safe as I travel," Eileen grunted, struggling with dragging her luggage as well as her suit of armor to the waiting car.

TIG couldn't stop laughing. "You'll never get through security in that."

"My good looks will charm them."

"Maybe. If they could even see your face . . ."

"It's going with me or I'm not going," said Eileen as she double-checked that her passport was handy.

"Fine. Suit yourself." TIG burst out laughing.

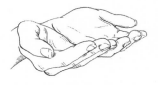

CHAPTER 7
Free Falling

Eileen walked through the airport to her gate. She overheard the song "Free Falling," by Tom Petty, as she passed a packed restaurant. *Thank you, Lizzy.* She remembered Lizzy's farewell message: "Deeply relax into the free-fall Eileen. The Universe has your back."

Her light shined a little.

She saw the sign for a Chipotle on her way to the gate and her stomach growled.

"Some food would be great right now."

ICK started in on her. "You're eating again?"

"Yes. That's what people do. They eat," said Eileen.

"That's what fat and lazy people do. That's what people

who spend money frivolously do," said ICK.

TIG interrupted. "It's OK to eat. That's what successful people do. They spend money on themselves to eat healthfully, and you are a successful woman."

Eileen stopped and picked up a quinoa bowl, water, and an apple.

A small piece of armor fell off. She noticed it, but because it was in a place where others couldn't see, she didn't try to patch it back into place.

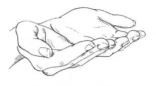

CHAPTER 8
Please Say Yes

Signs in Portuguese and English directed Eileen to the baggage claim, where Noella was supposed to meet her. Eileen's phone took a minute to turn on, but when it did she got a notification from her business email. Glancing down at the screen while she walked briskly toward her friend, she read: "Deposit into business account: $10,000."

"What?" Eileen stopped in the middle of the walkway.

She'd been awarded a business contract that covered her expenses for the next two months. She felt a mixture of excitement and confusion because she wasn't expecting it.

"Are you walking toward baggage?" Noella texted.

She couldn't push this gift away. The payment was already

wired to her bank account. She didn't want anyone to know, but she also couldn't help but feel proud of herself.

***

Noella's house was in Ericeira. It was a quaint fishing and surfing village, with a traditional town center of cobbled streets and whitewashed houses. The central beach overlooked the fishing harbor and was surrounded by sheer cliffs. A pleasant stretch of golden sand. Fishermen delivered fresh fish to the local restaurants.

One morning Noella shared with Eileen, "I want to move forward on writing two TV scripts I've been thinking about."

"Great," said Eileen.

"I'm going to pitch a few directors the next time I'm in LA. I'll get in touch with an agent friend of mine for ideas on how to make that happen."

"Noella, you showed me your painting room and your finished paintings. They are gorgeous! When you talk about painting, you transform. You light up. When you talk about writing the TV scripts, you're flat. What's up with that?"

Noella's paintings were reminiscent of the time Eileen spent strolling through art galleries during holiday breaks from college. In those quiet rooms, she lost herself in deep connection with the artists and their creations.

CHAPTER 8

"Writing TV scripts is what I've always done. I'm good at it. It pays the bills. Besides, you can't make a living by painting," said Noella.

"Have you ever tried to sell any of your pieces?" Eileen could picture Noella's painting of the ocean waves crashing against the cliffs of Ericeira.

"I wouldn't know where to begin."

"I can help you figure out a way to go after what you want. It's my specialty," Eileen explained. "It's what I help my clients with and they've gone on to do amazing things. I'd like to walk you through my coaching process. Please say yes."

Noella hesitated. "Are you sure?"

"Hell yeah!"

***

Eileen walked her through the step-by-step process and quickly refocused Noella's attention on the vital few steps to move forward. She gave her a plan of action to take.

Noella understood how her limiting thoughts and beliefs—that she can't make money selling her paintings—were holding her back. Eileen encouraged her toward a vision for her life, and showed her how to harness and uncover her deeply felt personal truths.

After the last session, Noella stood up and placed her hands on her heart. "You gave me a clear way forward. You built a meaningful and powerful toolbox that's unlike any other. You have remarkable insight and compassion that's grounded in practical realities and life experiences. I loved receiving your focused attention and active listening. Your method lives where strategy and spirit intersect. I am grateful to receive your gifts." Noella exuded gratitude and love.

Eileen knew she needed to take this in—to receive her friend's appreciation. She embraced her. "You are so welcome, Noella. Thank you for saying these things to me, it means a lot," Eileen said. Her smile was big and bright; she felt good.

"You let your light shine," said TIG. "Let it settle into your heart."

Another piece of armor fell off—because she let her light shine.

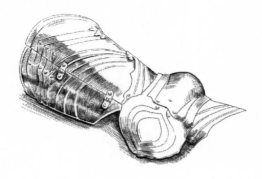

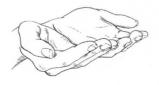

CHAPTER 9
Afterburn

Noella and Eileen settled into the porch lounge chairs with a fresh pot of coffee.

"I want my friends to meet you. They've heard me bragging about how talented and wonderful you are. It'll be fun." Noella blew on her coffee.

"It's too much trouble. Besides, people are so busy these days . . . "

"Not true, Eileen," said Noella.

Eileen muttered, "I appreciate your willingness to help me make business contacts. But anybody can do what I do."

"Really?"

"Yes, really. My skills aren't unique." She turned away from Noella.

"Your inner critic is brutal."

"I know," admitted Eileen.

Seagulls squawked overhead. The rising sun warmed the deck. Another beautiful day in paradise.

"Let my friends love you as much as I do, Eileen."

"Is there any other way?" asked Eileen, with a small smile.

Noella leaned over and gave her a hug. "Time to par-tay!"

***

At the dinner party, guests gathered around the kitchen isle, eyeing the inviting appetizer.

"Beer goes best with *ameijoas a bulhao pato*," a guest recommended to Eileen.

"Amia what?"

"Steamed clams. Get lots of *pao* . . . bread. The broth is the best part."

Chunks of garlic, onions, and sundried tomatoes clustered between the open shells. Eileen's mouth watered as she sprinkled her bowl with cilantro.

Noella wiped clam juice from her chin. "Not bad." Her eyes reflected the truth—her love of cooking.

Eileen let out a long sigh. *I do deserve to enjoy my life.*

"Eileen, by the way, this is my friend Bill. He works as a film location scout, he's touring around trying to find some sort of coastal charm town," one of Noella's friends said, directing Eileen's attention to a man who had just arrived.

"It's nice to meet you, Eileen." Bill extended his right hand, inviting Eileen to shake it while she returned the pleasantries. He had a warm smile that softened his eyes, gray hair speckled within the last remaining brown from his youth.

"So, what kind of movie are you working on? It sounds like a great job, traveling the world," Eileen said. Her hands were a little sweaty, and she couldn't help but feel her cheeks heat up every time Bill's and her eyes met.

"It's actually for a TV show about a musician, supposed to be from a Hispanic background, but the producers wanted a coastal setting, more like Portugal," Bill answered. "It's a great job. Getting paid to see beautiful sights, it's wonderful."

"I'm also kind of getting paid to travel. Not as exciting of a job as yours, but it's still pretty nice," Eileen responded. She and Bill separated from the party a little bit and stood close to the hors d'oeuvres. To calm herself down, she looked away from Bill and focused her attention on making a cheese cracker.

"What do you do?" Bill asked. Eileen looked up from her snack and met his eyes, which had been on her the whole time, she supposed, and felt her stomach twist. She hadn't felt this way in years, flustered by a man, but he was gorgeous. Could she even dare to think that he was being flirty?

"I'm a life coach for women. I have my own company and I help steer women back to their light," Eileen said. Bill smiled and nodded, seemingly impressed. Under his attention, Eileen perked up.

"That's so interesting. I think that's great," Bill replied. "I'm sure that your clients really appreciate what you do for them."

"I just can't believe that I've found something I love so much. It's important to me," Eileen shrugged.

The night continued. Eileen almost exclusively talked to Bill, learning more about his job and his trip so far, and she explained more of what she did. Eventually they got to talking about more personal things. Reluctantly she told him about her divorce, and he explained that his wife had died some years ago, leaving him alone with a young daughter. His kindness came through, and his devotion to his work and his family made Eileen feel light. She couldn't remember the last time she felt sexy, wanted, and interesting with a man, and Bill was making her feel all these things and more.

Eventually though, the night ended. Eileen left, but not before Bill gave her a big hug goodbye and a promise to contact her. While the prospect of further communication with the man excited her, she also felt sure that she was not ready for a romance. It was enough to test the waters.

When she went to bed, she drew and talked with TIG.

"TIG, I'm confused. I had a great time and now my throat is tight."

TIG said, "You're not confused. You're in afterburn. That's when you do something that is good for you— a new behavior—and then you feel off. Your inner critic says, 'Change back!' It's growing pains."

"You had fun," TIG continued. "You flirted with Bill and forgot about your worries. Give yourself time to assimilate this new experience."

Eileen continued to draw. "TIG, I won't be safe without my armor."

"You've never tried to go without it before," said TIG. "It's not dangerous. It's just unfamiliar."

"What's inside the armor? What if I don't like what I find?"

"There's only one way to find out."

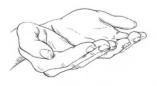

CHAPTER 10
Hold the Bitter with the Sweet

The next morning, Eileen walked to the beach to watch the surfers. Pine trees lined the cliffs and led down to the ocean. Surrounded by pines, the air smelled of Christmas. Pinecones scattered, the size of softballs. Locals ate their lunches on picnic benches.

The vast ocean opened up to her. No words. No noise. Only vastness. And a deep, grounded feeling that she was safe and loved.

She remembered her conversation with Bill last night, at first smiling, but then she started to panic. It had only been a year since the divorce, was she moving too fast? Could she just replace that love with another man? Was she betraying her relationship with her ex-husband? An intense urge to call her him came over her. They both loved the beach, which started from the very beginning of their relationship. They spent summers in a group house in Carolina Beach and eventually bought their own home there.

Instead she brought out her sketchbook.

A knot settled in her throat. "TIG, help me. Why do I want to call my ex? I'm in paradise. I'm living my dream. I met a new man. This is stupid."

TIG said, "You need to feel your emotions."

"No. It's going to hurt too much."

"Feeling your emotions will not hurt you but avoiding them does. Your throat tightening is a message from your emotions. Pause and notice that a strong emotion is present. Notice what is happening in your body. The recognition of your feelings brings you into contact with yourself and the present moment. Acknowledge and accept what's happening. You don't have to like it."

ICK jumped in. "It's why your ex left you. Because you were too emotional."

"I don't want to feel this," she mumbled. "Why can't I be over the grief of my marriage ending? It's been long enough. Why do I still experience moments of sadness?"

"Because you're human," said TIG. "And you have

memories. Sometimes bitter, sometimes sweet. There will still be times when you miss him. Sometimes you will cry over the ending of your marriage. It's OK. It is safe to allow these emotions to come up. Once they pass through you, you won't have to process that piece again."

Eileen allowed the tears to flow and her throat released its tight grip. She sat on the cliff and watched the surfers. She sent warm thoughts to her ex-husband. "May you be happy and healthy. May you be free from suffering and delusion. May you have ease of being."

"TIG, I don't understand emotions," said Eileen. She sketched angry faces and expletives across the page.

"Emotions tell you something about your needs, Leenie. They communicate what's going on inside you. Fear wants to protect you; anger means someone crossed a boundary; love signals that someone is important to you. Your emotions tell you who you are and what's important to you."

Eileen's hand paused. She ripped the page out.

TIG continued. "Emotions are meant to be experienced, and you aren't a bad person for moving on from your husband. It's healthy. You can't live your life in a memory, sacrificing your happiness for a bond that's already been broken. You deserve love and compassion, from others and from yourself. And you should engage in the Thawing Process."

"What the heck is a Thawing Process?," Eileen retorted, rolling her eyes a little bit.

"It's when you start to melt away the wall of ice built up from years of defense mechanisms and sacrifices of your happiness, and your true self is revealed. It takes the warmth of compassion to do so, and at the end of the day, you grow and heal, feeling the sun on your skin again."

"Compassion is a waste of time. It doesn't work," complained Eileen.

TIG chuckled. "That's because you've spent years practicing fear. Having the experience of love and receiving what the Universe wants to give you is what this travel adventure is all about. To teach you how to receive love and to remember that you have inherent worth and value."

Eileen dug her pencil onto a new page. "Why can't I tolerate it?"

"When you feel uncertain and you don't know where your sustenance is coming from tomorrow or next year, you start to control to feel safe," TIG explained. "You are learning how to be present in the face of uncertainty. You now have a few seconds of pausing between stimulus—external circumstances that trigger your unworthiness and self-doubt tape—and your reaction of forcing a solution, working harder, and neglecting your needs. You are learning how to allow feelings to come up without labeling them as bad or wrong. You have inherent worth and value. Lay down your weapons that harm you—the knives of self-hatred, self-judgment, and constant measurement."

TIG waited for Eileen to catch her breath. "When someone offers you help, say yes. It may feel like a sacrifice to give up your way. This is normal and to be expected. If you take away a sharp knife from a toddler, they scream. So do you. Ask to have them gently replaced."

"Replaced with what?" Eileen asked her guide.

"Acceptance. Patience. Inner compassion."

Eileen grumbled. "Inner compassion is a kinder phrase for self-indulgence. I've done enough of that for a lifetime."

"Inner compassion is a habit for those who want to have a great life and be successful in all areas of life."

"I'm afraid to receive," whispered Eileen. "I'll get body slammed if I do. My tools—make it happen/control/live and die by my to-do list—are what keep me safe."

"I know you've been hurt in the past. It makes sense why you don't want to try again. Can you have faith the size of a mustard seed today and trust the process?"

"Ugh. Fine. Just for today."

Despite her attitude, Eileen felt lighter and happier with the little mustard seed. She did yoga on the beach. She gave herself permission to daydream, collect seashells, and delight in being at the beach. She was present.

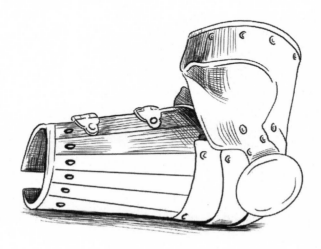

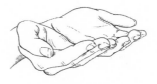

CHAPTER 11
Foreboding Joy

Eileen felt how good it was to be in Portugal. The food, the town, the ability to work while overlooking the Atlantic Ocean. She walked along the town's cobblestone streets, waved to the locals, and stopped to admire the fresh produce and pastries in the shops windows. One of the stores had the most gorgeous lace, handmade and hand-dyed. The technique had been passed down for generations. After days of reluctantly admiring the craftsmanship and beauty but forcing herself to walk past the store, today she stopped in and bought the one she's most drawn to.

Eileen remembered how rarely her mother, Anne, allowed herself nice things. She constantly cleaned the house, fixated on the appearance of it. Her prized possession was a lace doily her own mother had given her, and the kids were threatened with death if they dared to breathe on it.

Growing up, Eileen's childhood home was spotless. Anne worried about her kids all the time. She said the rosary whenever the kids left the house. She also cleaned when she worried. It was her way to deal with the constant tension in the house. It gave her a sense of control over the uncontrollable—other people, the uncertainty of what was going to happen next. Her mother worked herself into exhaustion, which led to bouts of depression. She would regularly end up in bed for a week. It had scared Eileen. She thought her mom was going to die.

Desperate for someone to talk to, Eileen called the only one of her friends who had ever met and gotten to know her mom: Lizzy.

"Eileen!" Lizzy answered. "How's Portugal, girlfriend?"

"Lizzy, I—can you help me calm down right now?" Eileen rushed out. "Please."

"Take three deep breaths and say, 'I am where my feet are,'" said Lizzy.

Eileen did this. Her breathing slowed down. She was calmer. "I am where my feet are." She stared at her feet, wearing sandals, bright pink nail polish, the sun shining on them.

Warm temperature. She looked up at the blue sky.

"What happened?" Lizzy asked once she's sure Eileen feels better.

"I just started thinking about my mom, her depression and anxiety, and everything. I can't believe she lived like that, and I feel guilty that I'm living like this, traveling and having a life outside of the house. She was never at peace."

Lizzy said, "Your mom lived like that so that you and your siblings could have a better life. She sacrificed in the only way she knew how for you. And it's OK to take advantage of that, so that your kids can have an even better life than yours. You are courageous— saying yes to what you want and releasing generations of shame and guilt from taking up space on this planet. You are learning how beautiful and generous the Universe is. It's as if you wore glasses your whole life and never cleaned them. Someone walks up with glass cleaner and now you can see in Technicolor. The light is bright. Your eyes have to get used to the brightness. Trust the process. Trust yourself."

Eileen asked, "How?"

"Be compassionate with yourself. It's OK to take risks and make mistakes. Enjoy this moment. Take care of yourself so that you can take care of others."

Eileen hung up and repeated her new mantra: "I am where my feet are. I am where my feet are."

Another piece of armor fell off.

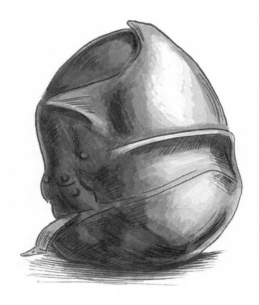

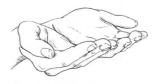

CHAPTER 12
Check In, Breathe Out

After a long afternoon nap, Eileen went for a stroll along the boardwalk. People were enjoying the evening, dining outside, shopping, strolling along the ocean.

Eileen noticed two women who stood frozen, like statues, in a doorway. "What are you looking at?" she asked.

"The sunset. Isn't it magnificent?"

Eileen turned around and became statue number three.

The sinking orange ball casted a beam across the water. Orange, red, and violet rays danced across the sky. Clouds lifted each one to the heavens.

One of the women released a deep, long breath. "Our yoga class starts in a few minutes. We have to go now."

Eileen looked at the sign on the door. "Sandhi House Yoga—Check In—Breathe Out. Welcome hOHMe."

"Holy cow," said Eileen. "I've been looking for a yoga class."

"We just opened last month."

"Great. I'll be back tomorrow morning."

The next day Eileen attended the class. The movements her instructor led her through at first pulled at her tendons and ligaments, stiff and unused to the exercise. It felt awkward, downward dog and sun salutations and the rest, but at some point her body started to move better, meld with the energy. The end of the class came quickly; Eileen felt loose and calm. A smile gently expanded on her face, and she thanked the instructor for a great class.

After some talking, the yoga instructor invited her upstairs to meet Liv, the owner of Sandhi House.

Liv poured Eileen tea and they told each other their stories. Liv had moved from Norway and, with very little money, opened Sandhi House. Their stories were both different and alike. They both were discovering what they loved to do and how to trust themselves.

Reviewing the conversation before she fell asleep that night, Eileen remembered one of her favorite quotes from Henry David Thoreau:

CHAPTER 12

"I learned this, at least, by my experiment: that if one advances confidently in the direction of his dreams, and endeavors to live the life which he has imagined, he will meet with a success unexpected in common hours. He will put some things behind, will pass an invisible boundary; new, universal, and more liberal laws will begin to establish themselves around and within him; or the old laws be expanded, and interpreted in his favor in a more liberal sense, and he will live with the license of a higher order of beings. In proportion as he simplifies his life, the laws of the universe will appear less complex, and solitude will not be solitude, nor poverty poverty, nor weakness weakness. If you have built castles in the air, your work need not be lost; that is where they should be. Now put the foundations under them.

If a man does not keep pace with his companions, perhaps it is because he hears a different drummer. Let him step to the music which he hears, however measured or far away. By doing so, men may find happiness and self-fulfillment."

Eileen smiled. She had taken another step toward what she wanted. The blankets pushed her body deep into the bed.

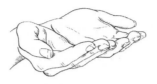

CHAPTER 13

Neither Good Nor Bad

Eileen woke up the next morning feeling wonderful. The sun shone through the white linen curtains, naturally waking her for the day. She rolled over in bed and opened her phone. Several texts and call notifications flooded her screen, the same words repeated: "Henry fell and broke his arm." "We're at the hospital now." "X-ray." "Doctor."

She tried to call her ex-husband: no answer. Next her oldest son, the only one with a phone, and he didn't pick up. Her heart pounded as her thoughts spiraled. Any calm she had achieved in the past days and weeks seemingly was gone, vanished, and replaced with fear and anxiety.

What was she supposed to do, an ocean and several time zones away from her boys?

Then her phone rang.

"Hi, Mom." She heard Henry's voice through the phone.

"Henry! What happened? Are you OK? Do you have a cast already? Are you still at the hospital? Can I talk to the doctor? Were you messing around again, how did you possibly break your arm, I can't believe it," Eileen was rushed, frazzled.

"I'm fine, Mom, I swear. I was playing soccer and I fell wrong, but I already have a cast—its blue! The doctor said it'll heal in a couple weeks. Dad bought me ice cream after we left," Henry explained.

"OK, honey, I'm glad about that. Can I speak to your father now?"

"Hi, Eileen," Rob's voice sounded gruff.

"What happened?" Eileen tried to not shout, but doesn't really succeed.

"He fell during the game, but it's OK, the doctor said that it'll heal well as long as Henry doesn't try to do too much too fast." Rob's story confirmed Henry's. She calmed down a little bit.

"Should I come home? I can leave right now."

"No, Eileen, it's OK, I have everything handled. I am able to be a parent, you know."

Eileen held the phone away from her ear and counted to three. "I'm not doubting that, Robert, but children need their mothers."

"Well, he loves you, but he's fine. We're all fine. You should stay in Portugal."

She wondered what he meant by that. Did they not need her? Was she expendable? Useless?

"OK, well, keep me updated. Let me say goodbye to the boys," she said, and then hung up once each of her children spoke to her. She looked at her phone for a little longer, reeling a bit.

"I need to fix this." She brought out her sketchbook, needing TIG's comfort, and drew a pair of wings, tattered and broken yet still trying to fly.

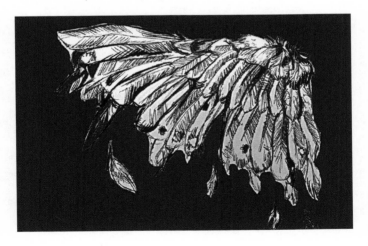

TIG said, "What if you didn't judge this situation—your son breaking his arm—as good or bad?"

"It IS bad."

"Everyone experiences in life things they'd rather avoid. Wisdom comes from being present under any condition. In every obstacle lies an opportunity. How you perceive a moment and what you do with it is up to you."

"I agree," said Eileen. "How I see this moment is that it is BAD."

"Have you heard the story of the Chinese Farmer?"

Eileen sighed. "No. And I don't have time for another one of your stories. I have to figure out my next move."

"It will only take a minute. Remember, you promised to stop being overly responsible and to learn how to receive." TIG shared the story.

A farmer had only one horse. One day, his horse ran away.

His neighbors said, "I'm so sorry. This is such bad news. You must be so upset."

The man just said, "We'll see."

A few days later, his horse came back with twenty wild horses following. The man and his son corralled all twenty-one horses.

His neighbors said, "Congratulations! This is such good

news. You must be so happy!"

The man just said, "We'll see."

One of the wild horses kicked the man's only son, breaking both his legs.

His neighbors said, "I'm so sorry. This is such bad news. You must be so upset."

The man just said, "We'll see."

The country went to war and every able-bodied young man was drafted to fight. The war was terrible and killed every young man, but the farmer's son was spared, since his broken legs prevented him from being drafted.

His neighbors said, "Congratulations! This is such good news. You must be so happy!"

The man just said, "We'll see."

Eileen's right eye twitched.

"Your experiences teach you not to lose hope or feel utterly defeated. Wait and see through all the pain and all the joys and say courageously, 'We'll see,'" said TIG.

Eileen blurted, "My experiences tell me I need to go home—NOW." She rubbed her eye. "'We'll see' sounds like a cop-out to me."

She remembered how calm and happy her boys seemed

on the phone, more excited about the ice cream than the fractured bones. They were OK. And they loved her.

TIG's advice was correct.

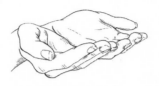

CHAPTER 14
Feel the Feelings

Eileen left her bedroom and met with Noella for coffee.

"Henry broke his arm," Eileen stated.

"How? Is he OK?"

"Yes, he's fine. Everything's fine. I still can't believe I'm not there, though. I know that it's OK, but I can't help but feel anxious. I guess I always feel anxious."

Noella said, "Does it feel like you're not on top of things if you're not anxious?"

"Something like that."

"I imagine it's scary to feel your feelings."

Eileen opened the refrigerator and grabbed the creamer.

What am I doing here? She poured too much cream in her mug. *You can't get anything right.* "Noella, if I could have my feelings bundled into an organ, I would have it removed. Emotions are confusing and messy. If I start feeling grief or anger, I'm afraid I'll never stop."

Noella scribbled. "Here's how I made peace with my emotions:

MAD + LOVE = great change

GLAD + LOVE = joy

SAD + LOVE = honoring

SCARED + LOVE = healing."

"If you listen to the guidance your emotions offer, you make peace with having emotions and experience healing, freedom, and change. It's time to make peace with your emotions."

Eileen knew this. *The longest journey in the world is the eighteen inches from the head to the heart* was what she told her clients. *What's wrong with me? Why can't I apply it to myself?* Her racing thoughts of actions she should take collided in her head. *I need to pause. And bookend my actions. How does the Animal Alphabet go? Ask for and accept help. Self-forgiveness. Hands-on-Heart. Remember your curiosity questions.* She rubbed her neck and screeched, "When am I going to get this?"

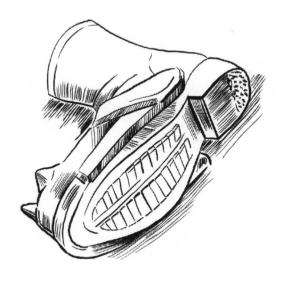

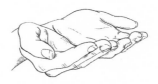

CHAPTER 15
The Big Guy Upstairs

Noella unpacked groceries from the farmer's market–kale, potatoes, sausage, and bread to make *caldo verde*. "I'm planning on going to Fatima this week, I'd love for you to come with me," Noella asked.

Before Noella mentioned it, Eileen had no plans to go to Fatima.

"I don't want to go there," said Eileen.

"I'll be with you every step of the way," said Noella.

"My throat is tight."

Noella smirked. "Sounds like your fear is trying to strangle you from discovering the truth about who you are." She rearranged the contents of the refrigerator to make space for the kale and sausage. "It's time to reconnect with your religion, or at least come to terms with it."

Despite the sinking feeling in her stomach, which she knew was reluctance and fear of how far she had drifted away from her religion, Eileen assents to the trip. She missed her relationship with God and knew that, despite ICK telling her that she didn't deserve forgiveness or acceptance, she wanted to have at least one talk with The Big Guy Upstairs.

Noella filled her coffee mug and sat down with Eileen.

TIG whispered, "Remember that pink and white Easter dress? You loved it."

Eileen's eyes, lips, and spirit all at once beamed. "Do they sell Krispy Kreme doughnuts after mass?"

Noella spewed coffee across the kitchen table. Her eyes teared from her uncontained laugh. Eileen grabbed a dishcloth as Noella assessed the damage.

"Sorry. I didn't try to make you laugh. I just remembered how much I loved biting into a still slightly warm Krispy Kreme doughnut after mass. Our church sold them as part of a fundraising campaign."

Noella glared over the rim of her glasses. "No. They don't sell Krispy Kremes at Fatima. Now help me clean up this mess you made!"

CHAPTER 15

"You talked to God a lot back then," mentioned TIG.

Eileen heard a child's voice. *I love you, God. I love that you made my dog Brownie and crayons, and my best friend Katie. I love my pogo stick and Krispy Kreme doughnuts. Let's draw together. You make me laugh.*

Her pulse surged. Happiness streaked across her face like a comet. She saw a flash of herself exuding a kaleidoscope of colors uncontained by her body. She wanted nothing else but for this moment to last forever.

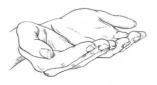

CHAPTER 16
Take It on Faith

The next morning, Eileen typed "Fatima" into Google maps and off they went. Eileen continued in her role as navigator and Noella as driver. However, this time Eileen started to feel carsick so she unplugged the phone and allowed the Google maps voice to direct Noella. She pushed on the acupressure points on her wrists, which usually stopped her nausea. It did nothing. Her hands tingled, then went numb. She felt light-headed. It had been decades since she had gotten carsick. She tried everything—windows up, windows down, A/C blasting, eyes open, eyes closed. Nothing worked. Shaking, she wiped her gray, sweaty skin.

Bile filled her mouth.

When they approached the Shrine at Fatima, Eileen yelled, "Pull over, now!" As soon as her hands and knees hit the ground, uncontrollable sucker punches lurched her forward. Eggs, banana, and coffee spewed across the cold concrete.

Still trembling, she sat back on her feet. Sweat stung her eyes and she wiped her face with her shirt. Slowly dragging in air, Eileen looked toward the sky. The leaves on the trees showed a million different shades of green; a Technicolor display of dazzling crystals—something she'd never seen before. She let her breath out with a deep sigh. "What is happening to me?" she wondered. "I'm losing my mind."

Noella brought her a wet napkin and water to wash her face.

Eileen got back in the car and the numbness in her hands went away. Five minutes later, the two parked and went to Mass.

During the service, Noella leaned over and said, "I was told that you getting sick before entering Fatima is a form of reconciliation and that Big Momma Mary wants you to receive communion."

"OK." Eileen sighed. "If it came from your source, I'll do it." Eileen took it on faith and received communion. Lightning didn't strike the church. It didn't fall into a pit of fire. She didn't get sick again.

On the drive back to their place, Noella hummed and sang. "You know what I think happened? I think you just

CHAPTER 16

released tons of worn out old stories and hatred toward the church. And hatred toward yourself. It was your body's way of telling you, 'Forgive yourself.' Now you have space for new relationships, love, prosperity, and joy."

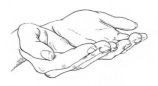

CHAPTER 17
Empty the Suitcase

Exhausted from her adventure, Eileen rested in a lounge chair on the porch, next to Noella. Sunglasses covered her swollen eyes.

"You said 'forgive yourself.' What did you mean by that?" she asked.

Noella smiled. "My mom would always tell me a quote by Norman Cousins. *'Life is an adventure in forgiveness.'* Forgiveness is not forgetting; it is being aware of what has happened and its value in your life. To forget injuries may mean you pass up a learning opportunity. Forgiveness is only possible when the pain that once controlled you is gone. The memory may last." She broke off a piece of a croissant and dipped it into her coffee.

"Most people have suitcases full of experiences of rejection, shame, betrayal, and humiliation," explained Noella. She dipped another piece of her croissant into her mug.

"Without forgiveness, you pack your suitcases full of these memories and drag them behind you. They slow you down and keep you looking backwards."

"I want to be free from all the stories I tell myself."

"Empty your suitcases," said Noella. "Ask yourself what you want: love, connection, success, fulfillment, friends, security...."

Noella brushed crumbs off her face and lap. "Give yourself a break. Forgive yourself for not meeting life's sometimes-impossible demands. Forgive yourself for not meeting your own expectations."

"Do I have to puke every time I want to forgive?"

Noella chuckled. "Hopefully not. The first step is to become willing. Are you willing to let go of the anger and guilt toward yourself?"

ICK interrupted. "Don't kid yourself. You screwed up. If she knew how bad you've been, she'd agree that what you've done is unforgivable."

Eileen was too tired to fight ICK. She asked TIG for help. "TIG—I can't take ICK's abuse anymore. I deserve better."

"I love you, Eileen, and I'm holding your hand," reassured TIG.

Her pale face told the truth. "Noella, I don't know who I am without those suitcases full of stories."

Noella beamed. "I do! You are a beautiful child of God. You need do nothing but accept your inherent worth and value. But you think you are the Prodigal Daughter who is bad and should be punished."

"Prodigal what?" asked Eileen.

"You know. The Prodigal Son story. I changed it to The Prodigal Daughter. The daughter of a loving father left home and *thought* she squandered everything for nothing of any value, although she had not understood its worthlessness.

"She was ashamed to return to her father, because she *thought* she had hurt him. Yet when she came home, her father welcomed her with joy, because she herself was her father's treasure. He wanted nothing else."

"Why is it so hard to believe this applies to me?" asked Eileen.

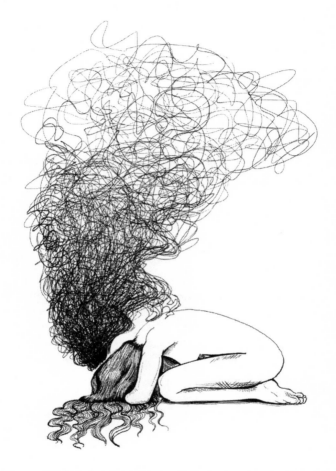

"Your negative thinking is why. We all have crazy thoughts. It's how we respond to them—or not—that matters. Are you ready to enjoy your life?"

Eileen rubbed her forehead. "Yes. Show me."

Noella explained, "When you give yourself permission to want what you want, you are saying, 'I believe in my inherent worth and value.' You make better decisions and choices that make you happy."

TIG joined in. "Relax and trust that you are safe and protected."

Noella went to her purse and pulled out a small medallion. "This is Michael, the Archangel of Protection. I want you to have it."

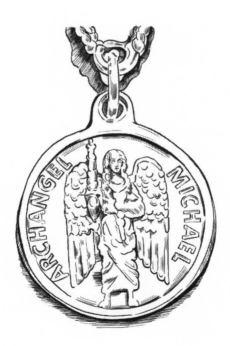

Medallion in hand, Eileen's mind flooded with forgotten memories. "I had a picture hanging in my bedroom when I was a kid. It was of a child angel on her knees. Every night before bed, my mom and I would say the Prayer for Protection.

Angel of God
My guardian dear
To whom God's love
Commits me here.
Ever this day
Be at my side
To light
To guard
To rule
To guide.
Amen."

Tears fell as she pressed the medallion in her palms and the memory in her heart.

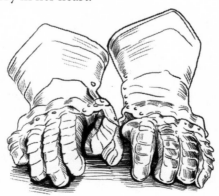

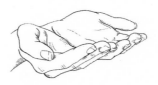

CHAPTER 18
Getting It Back

A gentle knock startled Eileen. "Good morning, gorgeous," Noella serenaded. "It's another day in paradise. Can I come in?"

"Yes. I'm still in bed enjoying my slice of it."

Noella snuggled into the overstuffed chair next to the bed. She noticed Eileen's sketchbook on the nightstand. "What's that?"

"It's my sketchbook."

"Can I look through it?"

"Sure."

Noella flipped through the pages. "There's a big gap in time between drawings here. What happened?" she asked.

"When I was thirteen, I stopped drawing."

"Why?"

Eileen grabbed her water bottle from the side table. "I started working. Walking dogs, babysitting, anything the neighbors would hire me for."

"You didn't draw after you finished your work?" asked Noella.

Eileen swallowed. "I lost interest in it."

"That's when you lost the light in your eyes," Noella sang. "Looks like Big Momma Mary is helping you get it back."

TIG started singing Joe Cocker's song, "You are so beautiful . . ."

"Dance Party!" Noella tapped on her phone and found her favorite song list. She pulled Eileen off the bed.

The world fell away and took with it Eileen's worries. Her body blurred in boundless twists and wiggles.

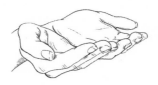

CHAPTER 19
From Stumbling Block to Stepping-Stone

Despite Henry's broken arm and the difficulty of the Fatima trip, Eileen felt better than she ever had. More relaxed, centered, and content in her body. Months ago, these setbacks would have crippled her.

"TIG, I've noticed something. ICK tells me it's selfish to go for my dreams. That if I tell you who I am and what I want, I'm being vain. Its favorite stab is, 'Who do you think you are?' I am sooo over it."

"That's ICK's favorite tool: shame. Its roots are in the past. You are strong enough to deal with it now."

"Shame?" Eileen asked.

"Shame means to cover. It's a normal human emotion. It tells you of your limits and boundaries and gives you permission to be human. When it becomes the core state of your identity, 'I am what I do, how much I make and weigh, how clean my house is,' it hijacks your identity. You forget that you are a beautiful child of God. Shame tells you there is something terribly wrong with you and that you are defective. Then it tells you to hide your 'badness.' That's why you work yourself into the ground, why you won't give yourself a break, why you won't give yourself permission to enjoy the present moment. Who are you protecting with your 'shame' identity?"

"My dad," said Eileen. "There was only one light allowed to shine in our family—his. If we outshined him, we were told we were being selfish." A memory bubbles forward. She was in tenth grade and did not submit her artwork for the school's annual exhibit at the town hall.

"That's why you protect the stories that keep you locked in your castle," TIG continued. "You're afraid of letting your light shine because you believe you'll get kicked out of your tribe."

"I don't want to be rejected by my family." Eileen cherished when her whole family got together at Thanksgiving. Each sibling brought their flagship dish and they enjoyed a somewhat friendly game of Trivial Pursuit.

"You asked me, 'What's inside my armor? What if I don't

like what I find?'" said TIG. "The seeds of your authentic self are inside your armor. You've kept it hidden and repressed. This fear of outshining your dad is keeping you stuck."

Eileen sighed. "Makes sense. How do I change it?"

"I wonder what you would recommend to your clients?" TIG mused.

"I'd help them write an empowering belief statement." Eileen smiled. "And that's exactly what I will do!"

Her pen scribbled feverishly. She looked up as though she just finished a test that she aced.

"Successful women embrace who they are and let their light shine, and I'm a successful woman."

"Yes, you are!" exclaimed TIG.

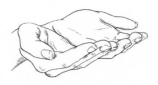

CHAPTER 20
Tormented or Free

"Have a great week and I'll talk with you next Tuesday." Eileen ended the Zoom session with her client. A salty breeze greeted her as she closed her laptop. She savored the view from her bedroom window. The sound of crashing waves reminded her of her new life. Sweet freedom.

ICK quipped, "You need to figure out how to pay Noella back for this."

I don't know what I can offer her that's equitable with what she's given me. Eileen's throat tightened.

"You have lots of great things to offer her, the most important being your friendship and love," TIG reassured her.

Eileen forgot all about showing Noella how to make a living selling her paintings. "I don't know about that . . .

maybe she would want a fancy bottle of wine."

TIG continued, "When are you going to set down your fear long enough to enjoy your gifts?"

"Enjoy my gifts?"

Eileen flashed back to watching her mother's anxiety. Her mom was anxious all the time—when things went wrong, and especially when things went right. Her mom constantly waited for the other shoe to drop.

Her mother struggled with receiving and had a closet full of tchotchkes, wrapped and ready to go just in case someone stopped by unexpectedly with a gift or to say hello.

TIG interrupted her thoughts. "Remember your mom's fur coat?"

"Ugh. Yes. She couldn't stand giving that present to herself."

Her mom had always wanted a fur coat. Growing up in South Dakota, she had a rich aunt in Sioux Falls who had three fur coats and wore them all the time. She boasted about them and how much money she had. Mom couldn't understand why her family was so poor and why her aunt's family was so rich. She felt ICK.

Eileen stared out the window. "Mom felt ICK too?"

"Yes. So did her mom. And her mother's mother."

Eileen's chest tightened. She imagined her mom as a child, alone with ICK.

"Remember when you won that Leadership Award a few years ago?" asked TIG.

"Yes."

"Do you remember what you thought when you were first notified?"

Her head drooped. "Yes," Eileen sighed. "I thought they made a mistake."

"Right," said TIG. "You couldn't tolerate receiving and letting your light shine."

Eileen thought about that day. Her colleagues hosted a party for her—cake, tea, and lots of love.

"You watched your mother do the same thing. She couldn't acknowledge her own gifts and talents. She hid behind your dad. His accomplishments were the only ones that mattered. Even after he died, she clung to his accomplishments. She hated spending time and money on herself. In a moment of sanity, she gave herself permission to want what she wanted—a fur coat—and bought it. She only wore it twice. She felt bad wearing it. Like she was bragging. ICK haunted her. 'You're too big for your britches.'"

Eileen connected the dots. "Mom couldn't let her light shine."

"That's right," said TIG. "Her ICK drove her underground. She was terrified to challenge ICK. She taught you the only thing she knew: hide your light."

"I feel really bad from my mom," said Eileen. *How did I not know Mom struggled too? I wish I could hold her hand and let her know how lovable she is.*

A ticking clock bellowed. The leather chair creaked under Eileen fidgeting.

"Let your light shine and break this cycle," said TIG. "It will not only release you from ICK, it will release your mother, and her mother, and generations of women who were afraid to let their lights shine."

Eileen said, "I feel even worse for my mom."

"Don't. Your mom is your biggest fan and cheerleader. She's rooting for you to succeed. Do you remember how your mom had angels all over the house?"

"Yes." One hung from the shower head in her bathroom. It was filled with lavender and the angel's halo was crooked.

"She knew they were there and looking out for her," said TIG. "That's why she taught you the Prayer for Protection—to make sure you knew you have angels watching over you too."

Eileen knelt down on the floor. Gut-wrenching sobs from her soul, filled with grief—for her mother, for her grandmother, for herself.

For the first time since her mother died, Eileen felt a connection with her. Like a warm blanket being placed around her body. She remembered dancing with her mom when she was little. "Shuffle off to Buffalo!" her mom sang as they tap-danced around the kitchen. Joy tugged at the corner of her lips.

"TIG," Eileen said. "I need your help to do this."

"You're already doing it. When you gave yourself permission and made the decision at 10:29 a.m. on March 22 to go to Portugal."

"What a coincidence. March 22 is my mother's birthday."

"I told you she's rooting for you!" said TIG.

Eileen wiped her wet cheeks. "My body is buzzing. What is that?"

"Joy," TIG said. "You are experiencing what you are. You forgot it at thirteen. Look in your sketchbook. You used to doodle 'I am JOY' all the time."

Eileen looked through her early sketches. *It's true–I did know this.* Her belly expanded as she filled her lungs–for the first time in years.

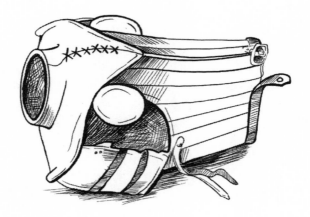

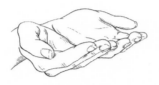

CHAPTER 21
Coming Home

Eileen drew.

"Keep going," said TIG. "You got this."

"Please help me. I need another mustard seed of faith to make it."

"I have something way better than a seed."

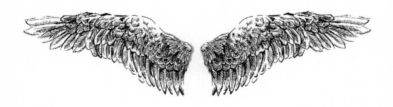

An image appeared in Eileen's sketchbook. Eagle's wings were spread across the page. Her make-it-happen wings rested gently on top, cradled and supported.

"Congratulations!" said TIG. "You learned how to receive."

"I did?," questioned Eileen. "I did!"

She jumped up. Her arms reached for the sky as she took a victory lap around the room. *I am finally free. Free to share my gifts and talents, to love all of me, and to let my light shine.*

TIG said, "Appreciate how your make-it-happen wings helped you survive until you could receive my wings. Love them with all the splendor they deserve. Thank them for their support, courage, and willingness to protect you for all these years."

Eileen wrote a letter to her make-it-happen wings.

Dear Make-It-Happen Wings,

Thank you for all your love and support over my lifetime. I appreciate your perseverance, resilience, and bravery. I see how hard you tried to protect me.

I want to apologize for making you do something that was not yours to do. I put you in situations where you got hurt, rejected, and abandoned. I yelled at you for being what you are—sparrow's wings. I starved you of love, appreciation, and friendship. I punished you. I abandoned you. Please accept my apology.

I promise to:

- Love you as you are
- Delight in you
- Celebrate you
- Include you on this journey of discovery
- Honor you always

You are now free to play, to delight in life's beauty, and to be my friend and companion on this adventure.

Love,
Eileen

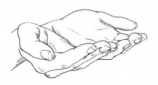

CHAPTER 22
Befriending the Monster

The screeching gulls greeted Eileen as she stepped onto the beach. The warm sand blended with her feet. She savored the smell of suntan lotion.

Her slow, deep breaths flushed her fears and worries out to the ocean. The sun's energy filled her body. Her skin glowed with healing light. She opened her sketchbook.

"I understand ICK now," said Eileen. "It's not a monster. It's a messenger. It wants me to love myself more, forgive myself, and feel all of my emotions."

TIG chirped, "The castle you built to protect you actually kept you imprisoned. You released it, brick by brick, and now have a new home full of treasures."

Eileen journaled about all the good in her life.

EILEEN'S TREASURE LIST

- I am lovable.
- It's OK to let my light shine.
- The Universe is a friendly place.
- I'm allowed to ask for and receive help.
- I have choices.
- Gratitude helps me keep going when I can't see my progress.
- I'm not selfish for wanting what I want.
- My emotions are valuable messengers and important to listen to and appreciate.
- I'm allowed to have fun.
- I know who I AM.
- I AM JOY.
- I am as God created me.
- I matter.
- I enjoy my gifts and talents. I gladly share them with others.
- I forgive myself for believing I was created unworthy and undeserving.
- I love my body just as it is, not as I think it should be.
- I trust that still, small voice inside me.
- I'm allowed to ENJOY:
    - The present moment
    - My gifts
    - My sense of humor
    - My body
    - Eating

- Taking naps
- Spending time with friends
- Dating
- Laughing at my quirks and shortcomings
- Balancing striving with allowing
- A mustard seed of faith is enough.

TIG piped in. "Now you know how to relax and love all of yourself—especially when you trip over your words or forget the reason you walked into a room. You love your sons with your whole heart and hold their hands as they learn how to live fully in this world. You feel your feelings when you mess up with customers and fail to close a sale because you are afraid of running out of money. You can handle the messiness of life without harming yourself. You are worthy of living a rich and delicious life!"

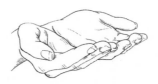

CHAPTER 23
Endless Miracles

"It's great to have you back home. I missed you tons," Lizzy gushed. The restaurant's music and patrons' voices hummed in the background.

Eileen looked over at the brick oven and saw it packed with pizzas. She turned back to Lizzy. *I have so much to tell her.*

"Lizzy," she paused. "I had no idea if it would work. I was terrified of running out of money, of disappointing my family, of ending up in an efficiency apartment alone. I had so many doubts. 'What are you doing? This is stupid. Nobody does this. Who do you think you are? Just go home and do what everybody else is doing. Get back to reality. Be practical.'"

Lizzy nodded as she bit into a slice of pizza.

"Every time I came up against an obstacle, the Universe rushed in to help me overcome it. The miracles were endless."

Eileen dug into her Caesar salad. *I love this restaurant. I love my life.*

"I closed my business books yesterday. There it was in black and white: the reality that it worked. Not only did I given myself permission to want what I want and go to Portugal for a month, I made enough money to support myself and my sons. And I didn't incur any new debt while traveling."

Lizzy raised her right arm and opened her hand. "Drop the mic! We do live in a friendly Universe."

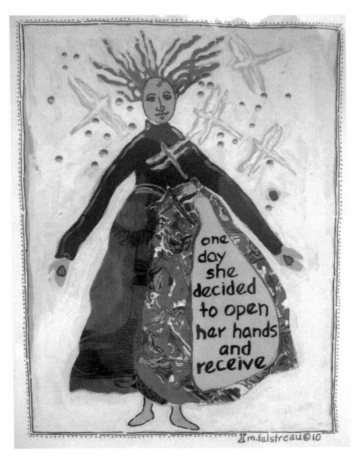

Printed with permission from the artist, Marylou Falstreau. https://mfalstreau.com/

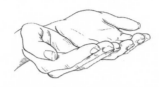

GUIDE TO RECEIVING
You Are Magnificent!

- Do you believe you are magnificent—without any qualifiers? A qualifier goes like this: "I'll be magnificent when I get that bonus, lose weight, or clean out my closet."
- Does it feel like bragging if you tell yourself you're magnificent? It's not, but it may feel like it is. Many of us were taught to put ourselves last and, as a consequence, we attract feelings of being unworthy and undeserving.
- Are you willing to change the concept of yourself? This means to be willing to change what you believe to be true.
- Here are a few ways to change the mental framework (qualifiers) about yourself:
    - Give yourself an A+ today in every area of your life. Does this feel uncomfortable?

It may, because you have a mental framework that you believe you have to earn the A+. Doing this experiment is one way of relaxing into yourself. When was the last time you gave yourself a break?

- Track your successes—all of them. I have one client who puts her successes on green sticky notes (the color of life) and pins them on a cork board. At the end of the week, she is delighted to see how magnificent she is. She moves them to a journal and starts the process over again the following week. A success can be saying no instead of yes, asking for help, speaking up, asking for a raise, or giving tough feedback.
- Allow yourself to want what you want.
- It's OK to have needs. They are neither good nor bad. Only your judgment makes them so.
- Write down the things and experiences in life that bring you the most joy. Look for examples that include: acceptance, creativity, intellectual, safety, simplicity, harmony, control, independence, freedom, challenge, connection, accomplishment, or contribution.
- Pause and give attention to the present moment. Ask, "What do I need right now?"

YOU ARE MAGNIFICIENT!

- Stop confusing receiving with taking.
- Expect resistance in the form of ICK. This is normal and to be expected.
- Accept the good that life wants you to have.
- For you is not against others. For you is better for others. For you is for them too.
- Find a guide(s) to show you how to go on your heroine's journey.

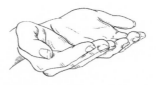

The Heroine's Journey

The heroine's journey describes a woman's search for wholeness. The heroine goes on an adventure, faces and overcomes a crisis, and returns home transformed. She confronts her dark side and emerges stronger.

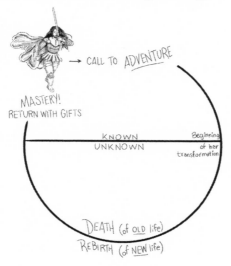

The journey is internal and circular, repeating trials and obstacles until she changes and grows.

Your heroine's journey is where you make long-lasting changes and return with gifts of increased happiness and peace of mind.

For Eileen, it began when she was challenged to go after what she wanted—a trip to Portugal. She faced obstacles along the way: self-doubt, misplaced guilt, over-responsibility, and ICK. She had a guide—TIG—and helpers – Noella, Lizzy, Rob, and Bill.

Eileen returned with many treasures: increased self-confidence, self-trust, and self-love. She let her light shine for herself and for others.

***

Each day, you are called to an adventure. Answer the call. Go into the unknown with friends. Embrace the unknown and stay on your path.

Accept support from your guides. Come back with treasures.

What do you have to lose? Maybe some anxiety, self-loathing, and exhaustion. What do you have to gain? Self-acceptance, increased confidence, and peace of mind.

Act as if you believe you are fabulous and magnificent. You are!

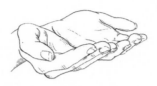

About the Author

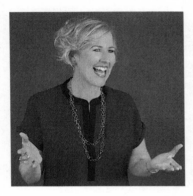

Moira Lethbridge, M.Ed., is the principal and owner of Lethbridge & Associates LLC. As a partner, strategist, and facilitator, she works with business owners, executives, and individuals to help them grow their business, do more of what they enjoy, and balance health, well-being, and achievement. Her expertise is executive coaching and personal development. She helps both organizations and individuals clarify their goals and achieve their desired results.

Previously, she was president and CEO of a professional services firm; she grew the company from 5 to 200 employees, increased revenue from $3 million to $35 million, and was named one of *SmartCEO* magazine's "Smart 100" in the Washington, DC, area for three years running. She is certified to administer leadership assessment tools including The Leadership Circle Profile (TLC), the Myers-Briggs Type Indicator (MBTI), and the Herrmann Brain Dominance Instrument (HBDI). Her services include business and executive coaching, strategic planning, mindfulness, and leadership and personal development.

She is the author of *Savvy Woman In 5 Minutes A Day: Make Time For A Life That Matters*. It contains 365 stories to help you balance health, well-being, and productivity. Invest just five minutes of the day to read one story and put the takeaway into action. In this way, you can achieve success at a high level. Find out more at www.savvywomanbook.com.

In 2018, Moira took a bold leap and traveled the world on standby to experience a life-changing mobile adventure. She discovered the world is indeed friendly.

The Gift of Receiving

5-Day Free Program

Are you successful and stuck?

Do you feel guilty or selfish when you take time to focus on your wants and needs?

Are you ready to live a rich and delicious life?

Receiving is a skill that you can learn, and it can be fast, easy, and fun!

Join My 5-Day Free Online Program

The Gift of Receiving: A Step-by-Step Guide to Release Shame and Guilt that Block you from a Rich and Delicious Life

If you are you ready to:

- Release misplaced guilt and shame
- Give voice to your authentic wants and needs

109

- Receive the gifts the Universe is trying to give you – mentally, physically, emotionally, and spiritually

Then this program is for you!

Benefits:

- Gain clarity on what you want and align your behaviors with them
- Define success on your terms and overcome limiting thoughts and beliefs that hold you back
- Learn how to receive in a way that is nurturing for you

It's OK to have what you truly want! Learn an approach to thinking and acting on the belief that there is abundance in the Universe, plenty for everyone, including you.

To Subscribe to the 5-Day Free Program go to:

www.giftofreceiving.com/5-day

or email 5day@giftofreceiving.com

THE GIFT OF RECEIVING

Made in the USA
Middletown, DE
21 February 2020